Your Free Gift

I want to say thank you for buying my book so I put together a free gift for you!

This gift is a perfect compliment for the book, it's a little bonus recipe you can use around your house!

Just Visit The Link Below And Download It Totally Free!

lucrativelifepublishing.com/free-gift-easy-essentail-oils

I hope you enjoy this awesome treat.

Thank You For Supporting My Work.

Sydney Summers

Table of Contents

What are Essential Oils?

Mankind has known for millennia that Mother Nature has a fully stocked medicine cupboard filled with healing plants and botanicals. Unlike conventional and synthetic medicines, the useful compounds and oils in roots, leaves, berries and flowers are milder and less toxic to the body and the environment in general.

By distilling a plant's sap or extracting its oils, we can concentrate the *essence* of the plant, making it more powerful. Essential oils can be prepared in many different ways, but each method is designed to extract a concentrated and purified form of the plan proteins and compounds that are useful in cosmetic and medicinal preparations.

The "essential" part thus refers to the aromatic extracts of the plant and doesn't mean that they are essential to health. But start using essential oils in your daily life and you might disagree!

The Benefits of Essential Oils

A single drop of essential oil is like drinking around 50 cups of tea made from that plant. In other words, the main benefit of using essential oils is that they are *potent*.

A pure, high quality oil delivers an intense shot of healing phytonutrients and plant compounds, and can be a very appealing alternative to antibiotics and other harsh medications.

Essential oils have a whole range of benefits for the human body. They can be used to treat infections, strengthen the immune system or lose weight. They can be massaged onto the skin or inhaled, added to bath water or diffused into the air to subtly alter your mood. In fact, there seems to be nothing that these little botanical powerhouses can't do.

Naturally, a big part of the charm of essential oils is how lovely they smell. In aromatherapy, different plant essences are used to activate certain mood states, encouraging energy, a feeling of wellness or even as an aphrodisiac. Of course, picking an oil simply because you love the aroma is great, too.

Alertness	Rosemary, thyme, peppermint, sage
Calm	Lavender, clary sage, roman chamomile
Sensuality	Ylang ylang, jasmine, rose, neroli, sandalwood, patchouli
Energizing	Lemon, grapefruit, bergamot
Focusing	Oak moss, vetiver, petitgrain
Uplifting	Vanilla, cinnamon, clove

Essential Oil Safety

It's a mistake to think that just because essential oils are "natural", that they are perfectly harmless and can be used by anyone in any quantity. In fact, some oils can be very strong and irritating if applied directly to the skin or if the fumes are breathed in or get into the eyes.

If you are pregnant or breastfeeding, be particularly careful and make sure that the oil you are using is safe. It's best to consult a qualified herbalist. In any case, try to do a skin patch test first to see if an oil will be tolerated, especially if you intend to use it in a topical application. Rub a tiny drop onto the skin on the inside of the arm and leave for 12 hours or so to see how you react.

Burnt or diffused oils are usually harmless but can cause eye and nose irritation in some people. Make sure that you have proper ventilation when using essential oils to avoid this.

A note on price and quality

When it comes to essential oils, you really do get what you pay for.

Many excited beginners will pick up any old oil from the drugstore not realizing that they have bought a product that has been watered down and adulterated.

When dealing with distilled plant essences in this way, it really is important that you buy an oil that has been extracted properly and carefully, stored well and not mixed with anything else.

Price is usually a good indicator of quality: a cheap oil has likely been pre-blended or is of low quality. A simple smell test of a high quality oil versus a low quality one will convince you forever of the value of getting oils from a proper supplier.

Some essences may have been extracted using harmful or irritating solvents, and some may even contain colorants and scent added, so read the label and become familiar with the seller.

Before you buy any oil, do a little research to understand the ideal extraction method (it differs for different plants) and be prepared to pay a little more for quality oil.

For oils that you intend to eat, make extra sure that you get therapeutic grade and not perfume grade, which may be toxic if ingested. Perfume grade oils are appropriate for massage and beauty preparations, although if you can afford therapeutic grade oils for everything, go ahead and use them for everything.

Later we'll explore some recipes that put essential oils to use internally, but because the oils are so powerful, it's wise to start small and work your way up.

What about flower essences?

You may see certain brands of "flower essences" being sold alongside essential oils in a store. These, however, are two different things. Flower essences are about the "vibration" and energy of a plant and are ostensibly captured in a tincture to be taken for ailments of a more psychological kind.

A discussion of the value of such preparations is not within the scope of this book, however it's important to note that they have very little therapeutic value as herbal remedies.

Essential oils are concentrated and distilled essences of actual plant compounds whereas flower essences are prepared by floating flowers on the surface of a liquid intended to capture its unique energy. If such essences contain any active plant material, the amount is negligible.

How Essential Oils Are Made

There are a few different ways that essential oils are created: using steam, extraction by solvents, distillation and expressing, to name a few.

Oils like lavender, peppermints etc. are oily herbs and need to be distilled. Water in a beaker-like apparatus is heated, and the resulting steam releases the plant compounds. This steam passes through a coil, which causes it to condense again, where it is collected.

Different plats require different kinds of distillation. Each distilled liquid is more accurately called a hydrosol.

Citrus oils on the other hand are created by directly pressing the rinds and peels of fruits like lemon, grapefruit and blood orange, just like olives. Another method is to use solvents like hexane for plants that don't have too much oil in them to start with, or otherwise contain delicate or volatile essences.

Other fats, waxes and resins can also be used as solvents, and the result is called a "concrete".

Another method is to use ethyl alcohol and then evaporate the alcohol off to leave the plant essence – called the "absolute".

As a beginner, it's important to understand how your essential oils are made and to what standard. What is suitable for perfumery and aromatherapy can be harmful when used as a medicine.

Where should I buy my oils?

Good question. Unfortunately, there is a lot of marketing and hype around some brands of essential oils, so much that it can be difficult to see exactly what it is you're getting in that little bottle.

Brands that rely on multi-level marketing schemes are not always the best quality and unfortunately, "therapeutic grade", "natural" and "pure" are not regulated terms. Some oils explicitly tell you that they are not meant to be ingested, but this could only mean that they are a small company and do not have the money to buy insurance that would allow them to omit that from their labels.

The truth is that when it comes to ingesting essential oils, your best bet is to consult (at first) with a qualified professional and see which brands they use in their own practice. When taken internally, essential oils are potent in any case. Taking poor quality oil can be downright hazardous to your health.

Nevertheless, here are some highly recommended stores:

Mountain Rose Herbs
Aura Casia
doTERRA (although some dispute the quality)

The Most Common Essential Oils

When you're starting out, you likely won't have the budget to buy a full set of essential oils. It's better to buy only a few of the kinds of oils you know will get used – this is also because the more specialized essences will be used less frequently anyway, are more expensive and may spoil before you get to use them.

Instead, opt for the most popular and common types of essential oils to start with. These are the most flexible and will have the most application.

A good beginner's essential oil kit

Lavender oil

Ask any herbalist or aroma-therapist and lavender will be at the top of their list. A beautiful, mild and incredibly calming herb, lavender has plenty of uses.

Bergamot oil

This gorgeous smelling oil comes from specific citrus grown only in a special area in Italy. It's also the ingredient responsible for the aroma of Earl Grey

Tea. A great oil for cleaning, perfumery and for its energizing aromatherapy properties.

Tea Tree Oil

Another popular and very useful oil is the strong smelling tea tree oil. It's used for its topical disinfecting and antibacterial action, and is great for treating viral infections and acne. A bottle in your medicine cabinet will find plenty of uses.

Eucalyptus oil

For colds, flus and congestion, eucalyptus oil is fresh and powerful, acting to unblock noses and chests when inhaled from a bowl of steam. Also very energizing and great for blends intending to help you "wake up".

Sandalwood oil

Good quality sandalwood oil is a thing of beauty. A wonderful, all-purpose scent for diffusing, adding to soaps and cosmetics and used in massage oils.

Essential Oils with Oil Blends

"Carrier oil" is a mild oil that other essential oils are mixed with. This is because essential oils can be too potent and strong to apply directly to the skin, for example. For massage oils or those that are burned in a ceramic burner, the oil will need to be mixed first with a milder oil.

The following are common carrier/blender oils:

Jojoba oil

This is an excellent oil to use for any skin-related preparation, as jojoba oil most closely resembles human sebum than any other substance on earth. It is incredibly gentle and well tolerated, and usually only a little is needed. Jojoba can be used alone as a facial moisturizer or hair treatment. Blend with a few drops of essential oil to massage or burn/diffuse.

Grapeseed oil and sweet almond oil

Milder, less odorous and usually cheaper than other carrier oils, grapeseed is thin, light and slippery, making it an ideal oil for the bedroom. Sweet almond smells light and fresh and is great for topical applications.

Olive oil

Providing the smell and taste of olive oil doesn't interfere with your recipe, olive oil can be incredibly nourishing and gentle.

Coconut oil

The medium chain fatty acids in coconut oil make it a truly miraculous ingredient to have in your home, regardless. Remember though that coconut oil can clog the pores if too much is used and though it's incredible for the skin, does take time to absorb.

Simple Essential Oil Recipes

All you'll need to start making your own blends is a few bottle of essential oil. It's also useful to have the following equipment, depending on the kind of preparations you want to make:

Pipettes
Spritz bottles for making sprays
A ceramic or glass oil burner with candles
Diffusing reeds and a bottle
Pretty vials to hold handmade perfume
Jars or tins to hold handmade lip balm or salves
Size "00" capsules if you intend to use essential oils medicinally

* Note: essential oils are damaged by exposure to sunlight, so be sure to keep your creations in dark or even completely opaque bottles. For the same reason, be wary of brands that sell oils in clear containers. Plastic containers should also be avoided as they may leech harmful chemicals into the oil over time. When storing oils, it's a good idea to rest the bottle on an absorbent surface like a towel or napkin as any leaking can damage surfaces, especially wood. If essential oils stain clothing, try massaging the area with a mix of baking soda and olive oil before washing thoroughly.

Essential Oils for Sleep

Lavender pillow

Fill an old sock with dried, uncooked brown rice and a cup of dried lavender blossoms. Mix in 10 to 20 drops of lavender essential oil and seal closed by hand or with a sewing machine. Now, when you microwave this pillow for two minutes, it will heat up and release a lovely calming scent that will last for ages if you store the pillow in a Ziploc bag.

Use on chilly nights to warm and soothe you as you read in bed, or put around the neck and shoulders to help the aches and pains from a cold or flu.

Calming night time balm

Mix equal quantities of chamomile and lavender oil (approximately 10 drops each) and combine with a half-teaspoon of bees wax and a half teaspoon of Shea butter. Mix together for a soothing balm that can be applied to the wrists before sleep to encourage restful dreams and to calm overactive minds.

Essential Oils for Energy

Here are the 6 most common energizing essential oils:

Rosemary
Thyme
Peppermint
Orange/grapefruit
Lemon
Pine

Used alone or as a combination, these scents in aromatherapy are valued for their energizing and stimulating effect. Rosemary is cleansing and refreshing and citrus fruits have been used for centuries to refresh, brighten moods and lift spirits.

Essential oils are so flexible you can use them almost anywhere, depending on your needs:

- Put a few drops in your morning shower or bath to wake you up. The lemon cellulite massage treatment discussed below will add to the effect
- Dilute a few drops in water and make a linen spray – as you iron your clothes, spritz with the solution to seal in a refreshing and clean scent (for bedding, choose lavender)

- Burn church candles and drop a few drops into the hot wax centre to release the scent, or else use the oils in a room diffuser
- A small bowl of water and lemon oil put in the oven on low heat will not only smell amazing, but the steam will help lift some of the grease on the inside of the oven

Warning: Be very careful with placing essential oils around the home as they can be poisonous to animals – make sure your cats and dogs cannot accidentally ingest them.

Essential Oils for Weight Loss

Peppermint to reduce appetite and soothe digestion

Peppermint essential oil tricks the brain into feeling full and is a great appetite suppressant. Burn a few drops of oil before meals in a diffuser or else sniff directly to take the edge off your appetite and eat less.

Peppermint is also excellent for poor digestion and is a treatment for all symptoms of irritable bowel syndrome and indigestion. Take a few drops in water with every meal to moderate the appetite and help remedy bloat, gas and cramps.

Grapefruit and lemon oil for weight loss

These essential oils can be used to lose excess weight, cleanse and detox the body and regulate the metabolism. Here, it is extremely important to only buy therapeutic grade oils – poor quality oil can do more harm than good.

Start slow by drinking, in the morning, one glass of water on an empty stomach, and adding to it 4 drops each of lemon, grapefruit and peppermint oil. Alternatively, the drops can be put into capsules and swallowed. Over time, you can increase the dose to 5 and then 6 drops of each, to be taken once a day.

Bergamot craving cure

Bergamot is a great essential oil for those emotional eaters and for stress and depression in general. Usually, cravings are a mix of stress, boredom, nutrient deficiencies or having too little quality fat in your diet. When you feel a craving coming on, quickly eat a tablespoon of coconut oil with 3 or 4 drops of bergamot oil.

Earl Grey tea also has a similar effect or else diffuse a mix of equal quantities bergamot oil and peppermint oil during the times in the day you know you're prone to bingeing.

Cinnamon tea to control blood sugar

It's no exaggeration to say that the way our body stores fat comes down to how healthy our blood sugar/insulin response is. Cinnamon lowers the glycaemic index of foods, regulates insulin release and can stabilize the metabolism.

After meals, make a tea of 1 teaspoon anise seeds, 2 drops peppermint oil and 1 drop cinnamon oil to soothe digestion and help your body use energy effectively, rather than storing it as fat. Cinnamon is incredibly warming and comforting. If it's too hot or you dislike the smell or taste of cinnamon, temper it will "cooler" herbs and oils like peppermint or hibiscus.

Essential Oils for Beauty

Home made perfume

Perfumery is an ancient and highly complex art, but with the knowledge of the simple principles, you can make your own simple perfume yourself. Your perfume can either be solid (set in a wax or cream base) or mixed into a carrier oil or alcohol. Each will smell different on the body, even if you use the same essential oil blend.

Alcohol evaporates quickly and so will create a "halo" of scent around your body, but can be drying to the skin and more transient. Oils last longer and give a deeper, richer scent, although only those close to you will be able to detect your perfume.

A balm has a similar effect and though it is the most lasting, will generally be more subtle. A good idea is to layer scents by washing with a scented soap, then layering on lotions and finally a perfume to create a more complex and multifaceted scent that lasts all day.

Any perfume blend must contain essential oils from three "notes". Base notes are heavy and thick oils, they last longer and have larger particles. You need less of them in a blend but they anchor and enrich the entire perfume. In some cases, the base notes are not even all that pleasant alone but can add depth to the other ingredients.

Middle notes add body and character, and tie everything together. Herbals and aromatics fall into this category. They add oomph and substance to a scent.

The top notes are experienced first in a perfume. They evaporate quickly and give you the perfume's first impression. Light florals or citrus fall into this category. Adding lightness and energy to a blend, they are tempered a little by the weight and longevity of the base and middle notes, but will disappear after a few hours.

Any good perfume will contain all three notes in a good ratio, generally an inverted pyramid (fewer drops of base oil, then middle notes and the largest portion made of top notes). Any blend you try will likely please your nose, but to create a truly beautiful blend you may have to try many, many combinations. After all, famous perfume blends are jealousy-guarded secrets for a reason.

Here are a few basic perfume recipes that can be tailored and adapted to your own nose.

3 tablespoons jojoba
25 drops of sandalwood oil
25 drops vanilla oil (a blend is ok)
20 drops grapefruit oil
15 drops bergamot oil

Floral bouquet blend

2 drops benzoin oil
5 drops cedarwood oil
10 drops lavender oil
10 drops patchouli oil
10 drops ylang ylang oil
10 drops bergamot oil

Dark forest blend

2 drops vetiver oil
2 drops cedarwood oil
2 drops peppermint oil
2 drops rosemary oil
5 drops juniper berry oil
10 drops neroli oil

Summer days blend

5 drops cedarwood oil
2 drops cardamom oil
10 drops lavender oil
15 drops chamomile oil
15 drops geranium oil

Unisex blend

5 drops juniper berry oil
5 drops sage oil
2 drops oakmoss oil
5 drops rosemary oil
5 drops peppermint oil
10 drops lavender oil

Old world charm blend

10 drops lavender oil
10 drops rose oil
10 drops lemon oil

10 drops patchouli oil
10 drops ylang ylang oil
10 drops neroli oil
5 drops clove oil

10 drops vanilla oil
20 drops rose oil
15 drops ylang ylang oil
5 drops sandalwood oil

10 drops vetiver oil
10 drops ginger oil
20 drops grapefruit oil

10 drops sandalwood oil
20 drops ylang ylang oil
20 drops jasmine oil
10 drops sweet orange oil
5 drops benzoin oil
2 drops lavender oil

10 drops vetiver oil
20 drops lime oil
15 drops sweet pine oil
20 drops rosemary oil
10 drops sweet orange oil
5 drops lavender oil

Warm and spicy blend

10 drops sandalwood oil
10 drops vanilla oil
10 drops lavender oil
1 drop cinnamon oil
1 drop clove oil
1 drop cardamom oil

The above blends can be adjusted depending on your mood. A good way to start is choose a recipe and then adjust the oils until you like the result. Remember to keep a notebook nearby to record exactly what goes into each blend. Keep in mind that all blends need to have the three notes, but use your intuition and preference for the rest.

Remember also that something may smell strange and overly strong in the bottle, but when applied to skin will transform and change. Remember also that perfumes evolve over time, so give a new blend a chance before writing it off. Try it in a carrier oil, diffused etc. to see how the scent behaves.

If a scent feels too claustrophobic and heavy, add citrus or a clear note like orange blossom. If your perfumes are evaporating too quickly, add more of the base note to anchor it.

Florals of all kinds generally do well together. Something that smells too cold or clinical can be warmed by adding spicy scents like clove, cinnamon or vanilla, and a smell that's too "hot" can be cut with a few drops of peppermint, pine or lemon to cool it down. Experiment to find a blend that's all your own.

The above blends can be mixed with a carrier oil of your choice, blended with Shea butter or bees wax to make a solid perfume, or used pretty much anywhere you'd use essential oils – for example a few drops on a soft cloth added to the tumble dryer makes everything smell heavenly. Don't put neat oils onto the skin directly as they will cause irritation. Instead, put into the bath water, diffuse or add to cosmetics.

Body oil

The good thing about making your own unique perfume blend is that not only can nobody copy the scent, but you can use your perfume anywhere. Add it to bath salts, room spray, burn in an oil burner or add tiny amounts to homemade cosmetics.

A drop or two can be added to scentless hand wash or shampoo, or use to refresh pot pourri. Body oil is a good way to layer scent and is easy to make. A good carrier oil is avocado, jojoba or grape seed. Shea butter will make a creamier body butter style cream.

Simply combine a cup of carrier oil with around 25 – 30 drops of your own perfume blend – more if your perfume is light. Do a quick patch test to make sure the oil will not irritate your skin, then apply after a hot shower to seal in the beautiful fragrance.

Rosemary hair rinse for shine

This hair rinse will leave your locks glossy and tangle free.

Combine ¼ cup of apple cider vinegar, 1 cup of strong brewed nettle tea, 5 drops of rosemary oil and 2 or 3 drops of lavender oil (if you want to add any other oils for a personalized scent, go ahead.) After shampooing, slowly pour this rinse through the hair –

the vinegar smell will dissipate as the hair dries, leaving it smelling beautiful and very, very shiny.

Rose bath salts

Combine a cup of coarse Epsom salts with 10 drops of rose essential oil, the best quality you can afford. Sprinkle into a warm bath for a very feminine floral experience. Any other floral scents can be added to created your own special blend – try ylang ylang, jasmine, lavender or patchouli. Dried rose petals or lavender flowers can be added for an extra touch.

Scented lip balm

Melt one teaspoon of pure beeswax with one teaspoon Shea or cocoa butter. Add to this one or two drops of red food coloring, hibiscus extract or beet extract for a pink color. You could also use a little mica powder from a speciality store to get a more intense shade.

Lastly, add a drop or two of lavender or ylang ylang oil to scent your lip balm. Pour into small jars and refrigerate to set. A fantastic alternative to chemical-laden lip glosses. Be careful that it doesn't melt in the sun!

In the shower, be sure to scrub your thighs and butt with a loofah or skin brush; when you get out the shower, massage with a mix of 1 teaspoon sweet almond oil and 5 or 6 drops of lemon essential oil. This will help break down fatty tissue and release toxins from the body. Can be done daily.

Essential Oils for Massage and Intimacy

Warning: The oils discussed in this section cannot be safely used with latex condoms. Be aware and be safe when using them. In addition, some oils may be staining and difficult to wash out of linen, so be prepared and lay down a towel for massages.

Massage oil

Coconut oil alone warmed between the palms of the hands is an excellent massage oil, but add 5 drops of ylang ylang, 5 drops of patchouli and 5 drops of rose oil to make a light yet seductive floral scent that will linger on the skin for days. To really set the scene, try burning a few drops of ylang ylang and neroli in a carrier oil in a burner while you spoil your beloved.

Sensual shower

If there's room for two, drop a few drops of ylang ylang essential oil onto the floor of the shower to create a beautifully scented steam room – put the drops off to the side slightly so the steam releases the scent; of course, don't put them directly under the water stream or it'll just wash away.

Essential Oils as Medicine

Because essential oils are just that – the healing essences of plants and flowers, they are quite potent and can be used to treat colds, flus and infections. Many essential oils are rich in the plant's natural antibiotics and are antiviral, antifungal and anti-inflammatory.

Thieves oil blend

Legends have it that some ingenious thieves devised a way to avoid contracting plague and so were able to rob those who had succumbed to the deadly virus. Once they were finally caught, they were told to give up their secret blend to avoid execution. Though recipes for this infamous mix vary slightly, they usually contain the following essential oils:

40 drops of clove oil
35 drops of lemon oil
20 drops of cinnamon oil
15 drops of eucalyptus oil
10 drops of rosemary oil

Combine all of the above. The blend can be taken internally by placing in small capsules and swallowed every few hours to treat a viral or bacterial infection, or else dilute the mix in water and use to disinfect surfaces when cleaning your home. The smell is intense but quite lovely, so a little can be used as a regular room scent or anywhere else you enjoy the scent.

Eucalyptus oil chest rub

Combine 5 drops of eucalyptus oil with a tablespoon of coconut oil and massage into the neck, chest, bottoms of the feet and shoulders. This will relieve congestion and stuffiness – if you have it on hand, rosemary oil can also be added, especially if you're feeling fatigued from a cold.

Thyme oil cold cure

When you feel the first signs of a cold coming on, take 5 to 10 drops of thyme oil in a glass of water and drink quickly. Repeat every few hours until symptoms subside. Thyme isn't pleasant tasting but if used before symptoms gain a foothold, can have you back on your feet within 24 hours.

Candida Albicans is a yeast –like parasitic fungus that can overgrow in the intestinal tract and cause all sorts of havoc, the most common being weight gain, indigestion and frequent thrush infections.

Three oils in particular are excellent at killing off the bacterial overgrowth. If candida is a problem for you, you may find that a program of essential oils will help restore gut ecology.

Daily, take up to three tablespoons of coconut oil, either eaten directly or in cooking. Also, in the morning and on an empty stomach, drink a glass of water with 3 drops each of clove oil and oregano oil – these can also be mixed and put into a capsule if the taste is unbearable.

Gradually, you can kill of excess candida – be sure at the same time to eat plenty of probiotics and fermented foods to repopulate your gastrointestinal tract.

Acne regime

Try "oil cleansing" – cleaning your face with either olive, avocado, grape seed or coconut oil to rinse away excess sebum and then using tea tree oil to treat individual pimples to disinfect them and prevent the spread of bacteria.

Conclusion

Thank you again for downloading this book!

Hopefully in this short book you've been inspired to indulge in the luxury of essential oils and the organic remedies for a better and healither life. Living a healthy lifestyle doesn't have to be hard, nor does it have to be expensive! The best part about making your own home remedies is that its all super affordable and you aren't wasting any product!

If you are just starting out with essential oils, try some of the simple recipes outlined here and gradually work your work up to more complicated blends with the help of a professional aromatherapist. Nothing can beat the sense of satisfaction that comes with working *with* your body in natural and wholesome ways.

Finally, if you enjoyed this book, would you mind leaving me an honest review? Reviews are so important for authors like me and it would mean a huge amount to me if you took the 2 minutes to write one.

I do look forward in reading your review, thanks in advance.

Also, if you missed your Free Gift just flip to the next page to get it now!

Your Free Gift

I want to say thank you for buying my book so I put together a free gift for you!

This gift is a perfect compliment for the book, it's a little bonus recipe you can use around your house!

Just Visit The Link Below And Download It Totally Free!

lucrativelifepublishing.com/free-gift-easy-essentail-oils

I hope you enjoy this awesome treat.

Thank You For Supporting My Work.

Sydney Summers